Instant Pot Recipes for the Whole Family

Quick and Easy Poultry Recipes

Gertrude F. Jackson

Sommario

Introduction

Considering the idea of diet in current times are based upon fasting, instead our keto split second pot is based on the extreme reduction of carbohydrates.

This sort of diet regimen is based upon the consumption of certain foods that permit you to reduce weight faster allowing you to reduce weight approximately 3 kg per week.

You will see exactly how easy it will be to make these delicious recipes with the tools available as well as you will see that you will certainly be satisfied.

If you are reluctant regarding this superb diet regimen you just have to try it and analyze your lead to a short time, believe me you will certainly be satisfied.

Constantly remember that the best way to lose weight is to assess your circumstance with the help of a specialist.

Enjoy.

POULTRY

Bone Chicken

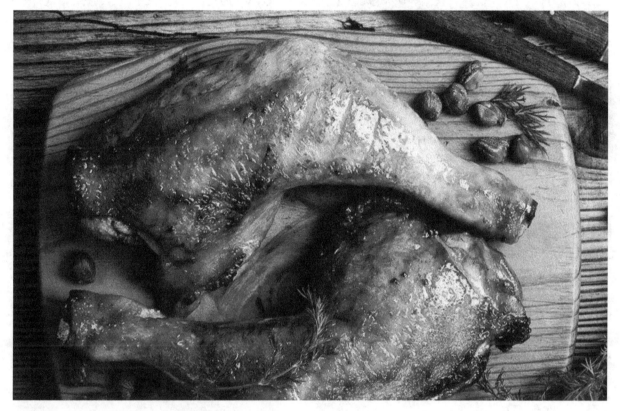

Ingredients for 4 servings:

1 tbsp packed brown sugar 1 tbsp chili powder 1 tbsp smoked paprika 1 tsp freshly chopped thyme 1 whole small chicken 3 lbs to 4 lbs kosher salt freshly ground black pepper 1 tbsp extra-virgin olive oil ⅔ cup low-sodium chicken broth 2 tbsp freshly chopped parsley

Directions and total time – 1-2 h

- In a small bowl, whisk together brown sugar, chili powder, paprika, and thyme. • Pat chicken dry with paper towels, then season generously with salt and pepper. Rub the brown sugar mixture all over chicken. • Set Instant Pot to Sauté. Once heated, add oil, then chicken, breastside down. • Sear chicken until skin is crispy, 3 to 4 minutes. Use very large tongs to flip chicken, then pour broth into the bottom of the Instant Pot. • Secure lid and set to Pressure Cook on High for 25 minutes. • Allow Instant Pot to depressurize naturally, then remove lid and take out chicken. Let rest for 10 minutes before slicing. • Garnish with parsley and serve warm.

Green Chili with Chicken

Ingredients for 8 servings:

2 tbsp unsalted butter 1 medium yellow onion peeled and chopped ½ lb poblano peppers seeded and roughly chopped ½ lb Anaheim peppers seeded and roughly chopped ½ lb tomatillos husked and quartered 2 small jalapeño peppers seeded and roughly chopped 2 garlic cloves peeled and minced 1 tsp ground cumin 6 bone-in, skin-on chicken thighs (2 ½ lbs total) 2 cups chicken stock 2 cups Water ⅓ cup roughly chopped fresh cilantro 3 cans Great Northern beans drained and rinsed, 15 ounce cans

Directions and total time – 30-60 m

• Press the Sauté button on the Instant Pot and melt butter. Add onion and cook until softened, about 3 minutes. Add poblano and Anaheim peppers, tomatillos, and jalapeños and cook 3 minutes, then add garlic and cumin and cook until fragrant, about 30 seconds. Press the Cancel button. • Add chicken thighs, stock, and water to pot. Close lid, set steam release to Sealing, press the Chili button, and cook for the default time of 30 minutes. • When the timer beeps, quick-release the pressure, open lid, and stir well.

Press the Cancel button and remove chicken to a cutting board.

Carefully remove skin from chicken and shred meat with two

forks. • Use an immersion blender to purée sauce until smooth.

Stir meat, cilantro, and beans into sauce. Serve warm.

Chicken Breast

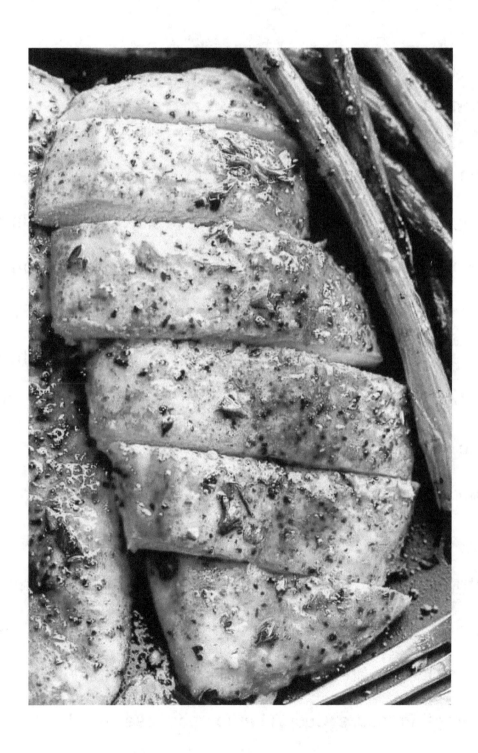

Ingredients for 4 servings:

5 chicken breasts 1 tsp salt 1 tsp pepper 1 cup water or chicken broth

Directions and total time – 15-30 m

• Season chicken breasts with salt and pepper add any additional seasoning to your liking. • Pour water or chicken broth into inner pot. • Place chicken breasts in liquid or on trivet. • Option 1 Fresh Chicken Press Pressure Cook/Manual and use +/- buttons to set for 8 minutes. Once the cooking time is complete, set the steam release to "venting" for Quick Release. If a crispier finish is preferred, you can swap out the pressure cooker lid for an Air Fryer Lid and cook for 1 minute, or sauté for 1 minute on each side. • Option 2 Shredded Chicken Press Pressure Cook/Manual and use +/- buttons to set for 10 minutes. Once the time is complete, set the steam release to "venting" for Quick Release. Drain the liquid and shred chicken breasts with forks. • Option 3 Frozen Chicken Breast Press Pressure Cook/Manual and use +/- buttons to set for 12 minutes. Once the cooking time is complete, set the steam release to "venting" for Quick Release. If a crispier finish is preferred, you can swap out the pressure cooker lid for an Air Fryer Lid and cook for 1 minute, or sauté for 1 minute on each side.

Chicken Risotto

Ingredients for 4 servings:

2 tbsp butter divided 1 lb boneless, skinless chicken breast or thighs, cut into 1 inch chunks 1 cup diced onion 1 cup sliced mushrooms 2 cups Kitchen Chicken Stock 1 package Creamy Sauce 1 cup Arborio rice ⅓ cup grated parmesan cheese 3 tbsp chopped parsley

Directions and total time – 15-30 m

• Melt 1 tablespoon of the butter in Instant Pot on SAUTÉ setting. Add chicken; cook and stir 3 minutes. Add onions and mushroom; cook and stir 2 minutes or until softened. Mix stock and Sauce Mix in medium bowl until well blended. Stir stock mixture and rice into pot. Close lid. Set Valve to Seal. • Select PRESSURE COOK (MANUAL); cook 7 minutes on HIGH PRESSURE. When done, quickrelease pressure. Open lid once pressure inside the pot is completely released. (Check manufacturer's manual for safe operating instructions.) Stir in cheese and remaining 1 tablespoon butter. Sprinkle with parsley and additional Parmesan cheese, if desired.

Cutlets with Tuscan Cream Sauce

Ingredients for 6 servings: 1 ½ lbs boneless skinless chicken breasts, cut in half lengthwise ¾ tsp fine sea salt ¼ tsp freshly ground black pepper 1 ½ tbsp extra-virgin olive oil 3 garlic cloves minced 1 yellow onion diced 8 oz cremini mushrooms sliced 1 tsp Italian seasoning ½ cup dry white wine ⅓ cup drained oil-packed sun-dried tomato halves diced 6 oz baby spinach one bag 2 tbsp chopped fresh basil 3 tbsp cream cheese or Two wedges Laughing Cow light Swiss cheese, room temperature ¼ cup grated Pecorino Romano cheese 1 teaspoon cornstarch 1 tablespoon Water

Directions and total time – 30-60 m • Pat the chicken breasts dry with paper towels. Sprinkle them all over with ½ tsp of the salt and the pepper. • Select the Sauté setting on the Instant Pot and heat the oil for 2 minutes. Using tongs, add the chicken in a single layer and sear for about 2 minutes, until lightly browned. Flip the chicken and sear for 2 more minutes, until lightly browned on the second side, then transfer to a plate. Add the garlic, onion, mushrooms, and the remaining ¼ tsp salt and sauté for about

4 minutes, until the onion begins to soften and the mushrooms begin to wilt and give up their liquid. Add the Italian seasoning, wine, and tomatoes and stir to combine, using a wooden spoon to nudge any browned bits from the bottom of the pot. Let the wine come to a simmer, then add the chicken breasts in a single layer on top. • Secure the lid and set the Pressure Release to Sealing. Press the Cancel button to reset the cooking program, then select the Pressure Cook or Manual setting and set the cooking time for 5 minutes at high pressure. (The pot will take about 5 minutes to come up to pressure before the cooking program begins.) • Let the pressure release for at least 5 minutes, then move the Pressure Release to Venting to release any remaining steam. Open the pot and, using tongs, transfer the chicken to a serving plate. • Press the CancelSauté setting. Add the spinach and basil and stir until wilted, about 1 minute. Add the Laughing Cow (cream cheese) and Pecorino Romano cheeses and stir for 1 minute, until melted. In a small bowl, stir together the cornstarch and water, add to the pot, and stir for about 1 more minute, until the sauce is slightly thickened. Press the Cancel button to turn off the pot. Wearing

heat-resistant mitts, lift out the inner pot. • Spoon the sauce and vegetables over the chicken and serve right away.

Chicken and Vegetables

Ingredients for 4 servings:

2 large bone-in chicken breasts about 2 pounds 1 tsp kosher salt divided ½ tsp black pepper divided ½ cup chicken stock 6 large carrots 8 medium whole new potatoes

Directions and total time – 15-30 m

• Season the chicken breasts with ½ teaspoon salt and ¼ teaspoon pepper. • Pour the stock into the inner pot and then add the chicken breasts. Place the carrots and potatoes on top of the chicken and season them with the rest of the salt and pepper. Secure the lid. • Press the Manual or Pressure Cook button and adjust the time to 15 minutes. • When the timer beeps, let pressure release naturally until float valve drops and then unlock lid. • Transfer to plates to serve and spoon the juices on top.

Chicken Soup

Ingredients for 6 servings:

6 cups chicken broth 6 oz tomato paste (1 can) 1 lb boneless, skinless chicken breasts 15.25 oz corn (1 can) drained 14.5 oz black beans (1 can) rinsed and drained 14 oz mild diced green chilies (2 cans) 1 tsp salt ¼ tsp black pepper ¼ cup cilantro roughly chopped

Directions and total time – 15-30 m

• Pour broth into Instant Pot. Whisk tomato paste into broth. • Add in chicken breasts, corn, beans, green chilies, salt, and pepper. Stir to combine. • Close lid and set pressure release to Sealing. • Press Manual or Pressure Cook button and adjust time to 15 minutes. • When the timer beeps, allow pressure to release naturally for 10 minutes and then quick release remaining pressure. Unlock lid and remove it. • Remove the chicken. Shred the chicken using two forks and then place it back into Instant Pot. • Serve soup topped with tortilla chips and cilantro.

Turkey Meatballs

Ingredients for 4-6 servings:

Meatball Mixture: 1 lb ground turkey ⅓ cup panko breadcrumbs 1 egg 1 tsp onion powder 1 tsp kosher salt ½ tsp pepper 1 tbsp Buffalo-style hot sauce Other Ingredients: 1 tbsp olive oil ¼ cup chicken broth ½ cup Buffalo-style hot sauce ranch or blue cheese dressing, blue cheese crumbles and/or thinly sliced green onions for serving

Directions and total time – 30-60 m

• In a medium bowl combine Meatball Mixture ingredients. Using wet hands to prevent sticking, form into 18 meatballs. • Add olive oil to the Instant Pot. Using the display panel select the SAUTE function. • When oil gets hot, brown the meatballs on 3 sides, 2-3 minutes per side. Meat will not be cooked through. Do not crowd the pot--you may have to work in batches. Transfer browned meatballs to a shallow dish and cover loosely with foil. • Add broth to the pot and deglaze by using a wooden spoon to scrape the brown bits from the bottom of the pot. Stir in the ½ cup hot sauce. • Put the meatballs back into the pot, turning once to coat. • Turn the pot off by selecting CANCEL, then secure the lid, making sure the vent is closed. • Using the display panel select the MANUAL function. Use the +/- keys and program the Instant Pot for 5 minutes. • When the time is up, quick-release the remaining pressure. • Serve hot, garnished with ranch or blue cheese dressing, blue cheese crumbles and/or thinly sliced green onions. • choice of toppings such as tzatziki sauce, sliced cucumbers, chopped tomatoes, hummus, olives.

Turkey Meatballs and Rice

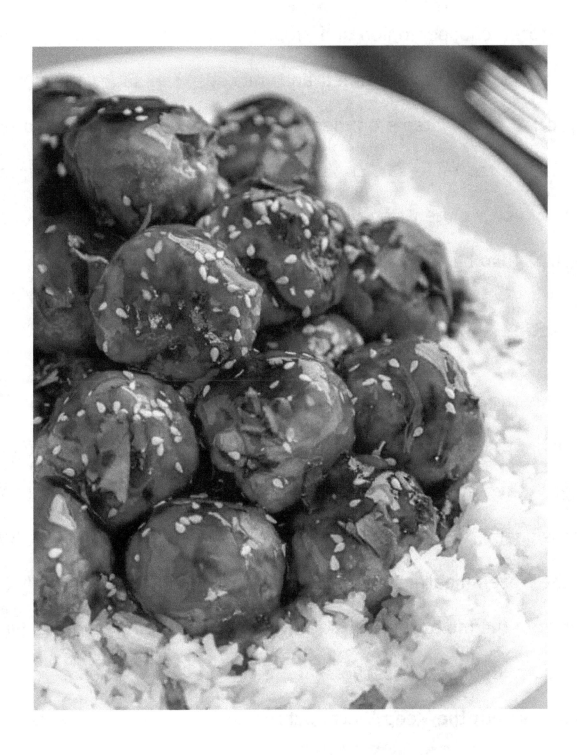

Ingredients for 4 servings:

2 ½ cups chicken broth 1 cup raw white basmati rice plus 1 tbsp ½ cup frozen chopped onion or 1 small yellow or white onion; peeled and chopped 2 tsp stemmed and minced fresh sage leaves or 1 tsp dried sage 1 tsp stemmed fresh thyme leaves or ½ tsp dried thyme ½ tsp table salt 1 ½ lbs frozen mini or bite-sized turkey meatballs (a gluten-free version if that's a concern), ½-1 ounce each 2 tbsp butter

Directions and total time – 30-60 m

• Press the button SAUTÉ and set it for HIGH, MORE, or CUSTOM 400°F. Set the timer for 10 minutes. • Mix the broth, rice, onion, sage, thyme, and salt in an Instant Pot. Cook, stirring occasionally, until many wisps of steam rise from the liquid. Stir in the frozen meatballs, then turn off the SAUTÉ function. Set the butter in the mixture and lock the lid onto the pot. • Option 1 Max Pressure Cooker Press Pressure cook on Max pressure for 10 minutes with the Keep Warm setting off. • Option 2 All Pressure

Cookers Press Poultry, Pressure cook or Manual and set for High pressure for 12 minutes with the Keep Warm setting off. • Use the quick-release method to bring the pot's pressure back to normal— but do not open the lid. Leave the pot undisturbed for 10 minutes after the pressure has been released. Unlatch the lid and open the cooker. Stir well before serving.

Teriyaki Chicken

Ingredients for 6 servings:

¾ cup chicken broth ½ cup regular or reduced-sodium soy sauce or tamari ½ cup frozen chopped onion or 1 small yellow or white onion peeled and chopped 3 tbsp light brown sugar 2 tbsp fresh ginger peeled and minced 1 tbsp garlic peeled and minced 3 lbs frozen boneless skinless chicken thighs

Directions and total time – 30-60 m

• Mix the broth, soy sauce or tamari, onion, brown sugar, ginger, and garlic in an Instant Pot. Add the block or hunks of frozen chicken, stir well, and lock the lid onto the pot. • Optional 1 Max Pressure Cooker Press Pressure cook on Max pressure for 17 minutes with the Keep Warm setting off. • Optional 2 All Pressure Cookers Press Poultry, Pressure cook or Manual on High pressure for 20 minutes with the Keep Warm setting off. • When the machine has finished cooking, turn it off and let its pressure return to normal naturally, about 25 minutes. Unlatch the lid and open the cooker. Use tongs or a slotted spoon to transfer the chicken thighs to a bowl. ● Press the button for SAUTE. Set it for HIGH, MORE or CUSTOM 400°F. Set the time for 15 minutes and if necessary, press START. ● Bring the sauce in the pot to a boil, stirring often. Continue boiling, stirring more and more frequently until almost constantly, until the sauce is a thick glaze, about 7 minutes. Turn off the SAUTÉ function. Return the chicken thighs and any juices to the cooker. Stir until the chicken is coated in the glaze. Transfer the pieces to a serving platter or plates.

Chicken with Cordon Bleu

Ingredients for 4 servings: ½ cup chicken broth 2 lbs chicken breasts about 4 chicken breasts 1 tbsp butter melted 2 oz thinly sliced ham 2 oz swiss or provolone cheese kosher salt pepper 1 tbsp olive oil 1 tbsp butter 1 cup panko bread crumbs 2 tbsp Dijon mustard 2 tbsp heavy cream snipped chives for garnish

Directions and total time – 15-30 m • Pour chicken broth into the Instant Pot. • Place chicken breasts, smooth side down, between two sheets of plastic wrap and pound to ¼ inch thickness. • Brush melted butter evenly over chicken breasts, followed by ham and cheese. Sprinkle with salt and pepper to taste. • Roll up each chicken breast starting at one of the short ends. Place each chicken bundle seam side down in the Instant Pot, then secure the lid, making sure the vent is closed. • Using the display panel select the MANUAL or PRESSURE COOK function. Use the +/- keys and program the Instant Pot for 5 minutes. • When the time is up, let the pressure naturally release for 5 minutes, then quick-release the remaining pressure. •

Meanwhile, heat olive oil and butter in a nonstick skillet. When butter is melted, add panko, ¼ tsp salt and several grinds of pepper. • Cook, stirring constantly, until crumbs turn golden brown, then remove from heat immediately and continue to stir for 30 seconds to avoid burning. • In a small bowl, combine dijon and cream. Set aside. • When cooking cycle is complete, carefully remove the roll-ups from the pot, dip each in the skillet to coat the bottom with toasted crumbs, then place on individual serving plates. • Sprinkle remaining toasted crumbs over the top of the roll-ups, drizzle with dijon and top with snipped chives.

Soup with Chicken and Lime

Ingredients for 2-4 servings:

1 tbsp olive oil extra virgin ½ medium yellow onion roughly chopped 1 stalk celery trimmed and roughly chopped ½ medium jalapeno roughly chopped 2 cloves garlic 8 oz chicken breast roughly chopped 3 cups chicken broth 7 oz diced tomatoes with chiles ½ can (14 oz) ½ tsp dried oregano ½ tsp cumin 1 tsp kosher or sea salt 3 tbsp Cilantro leaves 1 lime juiced

Directions and total time – 15-30 m

• Add all ingredients except the cilantro and lime to the blender pitcher and secure lid. • Select "Soup 1" setting • When soup is finished cooking, add cilantro and lime to pitcher. • Select "Low" setting and blend for three seconds. Select "Cancel" to stop blending.

Best Teriyaki Chicken

Ingredients for 6 servings:

2 tablespoons vegetable oil 6 chicken thighs skin and visible fat removed ½ cup apricot pineapple jam 2 tablespoons soy sauce 1 cup Water

Directions and total time – 30-60 m

• Turn Instant Pot to High Sauté and let heat for a few minutes. Add oil. Add 3 of the chicken thighs to the pot and cook until golden brown, about 3 minutes on each side. Repeat with remaining thighs. Press Cancel. • In a medium bowl, whisk together the jam and soy sauce and toss in the thighs until well coated. Pour water into the pot. Place the wire trivet in the pot and arrange thighs on top of trivet. Press Cancel. Place lid on pot and lock into place to seal. Pressure Cook or Manualon High Pressure for 20 minutes. Let sit for 10 minutes. Use Quick Pressure Release. • Remove thighs to a serving plate. Press Cancel. Turn pot to High Sauté and let liquid simmer and thicken for about 5 minutes, whisking frequently. Drizzle thickened sauce over chicken, to serve.

Chicken Pozole

Ingredients for 8 servings:

3 pounds boneless chicken breasts or thighs cut into large chunks 1 medium onion halved 3 cloves garlic minced 4 sprigs cilantro 29 oz white hominy 1 can drained, 3 cups Spicy Salsa Verde 2 cups chicken broth ½ tsp coarse salt plus more for seasoning (optional) ½ tsp crushed dried Mexican oregano Chopped red onion for garnish Shredded cabbage or lettuce for garnish Sliced radishes for garnish freshly squeezed lime juice for garnish Tostada shells or tortilla chips for serving (optional)

Directions and total time – 30-60 m

• In the Instant Pot, combine the chicken, onion, garlic, cilantro, hominy, and salsa verde. Add the chicken broth, salt, oregano, and 3 cups water. • Lock the lid into place and set the steam release valve to sealed. Select Manual or Pressure Cook and set the timer for 20 minutes on high. • When cooking is complete, allow the pressure to release naturally. Unlock and remove the lid. • Season the pozole with more salt, if necessary. Ladle into bowls and garnish with chopped onion, shredded cabbage, sliced radishes, and a squeeze of fresh lime juice. Serve with tostada shells or tortilla chips (if desired).

Chicken Salad in Envelopes

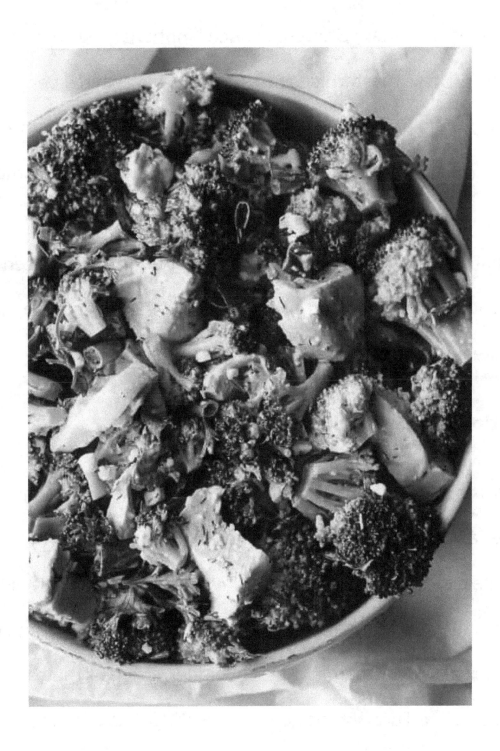

Ingredients for 4 servings:

Sauce Mixture: ¼ cup Hoisin Sauce 3 tbsp soy sauce 1 tbsp rice wine vinegar 1 tsp Sriracha sauce (optional) 1 tsp mustard powder 1 tsp toasted sesame oil ¼ tsp white pepper Pot Mixture: 1 tbsp olive oil 1 cup onions finely diced 1 lb ground chicken (or turkey) 3 cloves garlic minced 1 ½ inch fresh ginger piece, minced To Finish: 1 cup shredded carrots 8 ounce water chestnuts 1 can drained and diced 2-3 green onions green parts only, sliced thin 1 head butter lettuce, bibb, or boston, leaves separated

Directions and total time – 15-30 m

• In a medium bowl, mix together all Sauce Mixture ingredients and set aside. • Add olive oil to the Instant Pot. Using the display panel select the SAUTE function. • When oil gets hot, add the onions and ground meat. Cook and stir until no pink remains. • Drain out all liquid, then add garlic, ginger and half the sauce. Stir to combine. • Turn the pot off by selecting CANCEL, then secure the lid, making sure the vent is closed. • Using the display panel select the MANUAL or PRESSURE COOK function. Use the +/- keys and program the Instant Pot for 0 minutes. • When the time is up, let the pressure naturally release for 10 minutes, then quick-release the remaining pressure. • Stir and then drain out any remaining liquid. Add remaining sauce and stir to warm through, returning to SAUTE as needed. • Turn the pot off by selecting CANCEL, then add the carrot, water chestnuts, green onions and toasted sesame oil. • Serve warm with lettuce leaves on the side. Scoop a few tablespoons of chicken mixture into a lettuce leaf, roll and eat.

Seared Chicken Breasts

Ingredients for 4 servings:

2 tbsp solid or liquid fat. Choose from butter, lard, rendered bacon fat, schmaltz, or an oil of almost any sort: olive, avocado, vegetable, corn, canola, safflower, grape seed, walnut, almond, or pecan — or a 50/50 combo of a solid fat and a liquid fat. 4 boneless, skinless chicken breasts 10-12 ounces each 2 tbsp dried herbs or a seasoning blend. Choose at least two or many to make up the total amount from any dried herb like thyme, oregano, or parsley; ground cinnamon, ground dried ginger, or ground dried turmeric; a curry powder of any sort, herbes de Provence, or any dried spice seasoning blend from Cajun to Italian, French to Greek. ½ tsp table salt optional 1 ½ cups liquid. Choose from water, broth of any sort, beer, wine of any sort, dry vermouth, dry sherry, unsweetened apple cider, unsweetened pear nectar, or a 50/50 combo of water or broth and wine.

Directions and total time – 15-30 m

• Press Saute, set time for 15 minutes. • Melt the fat or warm the oil in the cooker. Season the chicken breasts with the dried herbs or seasoning blend and salt (if using). Set 2 breasts in the pot and brown well, turning once, about 6 minutes. Transfer these to a nearby plate and brown the other 2 breasts in the same way before getting them onto the plate. • Turn off the SAUTÉ function. Set a heat- and pressure-safe trivet in the pot. Pour in the liquid. Set all the chicken breasts on the trivet, overlapping thick ends over thin ends as necessary. Lock the lid onto the pot. • Optional 1 Max Pressure Cooker Press Pressure cook on Max pressure for 6 minutes with the Keep Warm setting off. • Optional 2 All Pressure Cookers Press Meat/Stew or Pressure cook (Manual) on High pressure for 8 minutes with the Keep Warm setting off. • Use the quick-release method to bring the pot's pressure back to normal — but do not open the cooker. Set it aside for 3 minutes with the valve open but the cooker off. Unlatch the lid and open the pot. Serve at once.

Peanut Chicken

Ingredients for 6 servings:

3 tbsp vegetable oil divided 1 cup raw peanuts 3 dried red chiles 1 tbsp cumin seeds 1 tbsp coriander seeds 10 curry leaves torn into pieces 2 tsp kosher salt divided 2 tbsp tamarind concentrate Water 2 onions diced 1 tbsp Ginger minced 1 tbsp garlic minced 1 lbs chicken thighs cut into 1 inch pieces

Directions and total time – 30-60 m

• Using the Sauté function on High, heat 1 tablespoon oil in the inner pot for about 1 minute, until shimmering. Add the peanuts and cook for 1 minute, stirring frequently, until fragrant. Add the chilies, cumin seeds, coriander seeds and curry leaves; cook for 1 minute, until fragrant. Transfer the nuts and spices to a blender and let cool slightly. Remove ¼ cup of the peanut mixture and set aside until step 4. Add 1 teaspoon salt and the tamarind concentrate to the blender; blend on high speed until smooth, adding 1 tablespoon water if needed to help the mixture blend. •

Using the Sauté function on High, heat 2 tablespoons oil in the inner pot for about 1 minute, until shimmering. Add the onions and cook for about 4 minutes, stirring occasionally, until softened. Add the ginger and garlic; cook for about 1 minute, until fragrant. • Stir in the chicken, ½ cup water, peanut chutney and remaining 1 teaspoon salt. Secure the lid and cook on high pressure for 8 minutes. • Once the cooking is complete, let the pressure release naturally for 10 minutes, then quickrelease the remaining pressure. Transfer the curry to a platter. Pour the reserved peanuts and spices over the chicken and serve.

Tagine with Chicken and Olive

Ingredients for 4 servings:

2 teaspoon sweet paprika 1 ½ teaspoons ground cumin 1 teaspoon ground turmeric ½ teaspoon ground ginger ½ teaspoon ground cinnamon 4 large chicken thighs skin-on and bone-in (2 ½ pounds to 3 pounds) Salt and pepper 2 tablespoons canola or grapeseed oil 1 onion sliced 6 cloves garlic smashed 2 tablespoons tomato paste 1 cup chicken broth ½ lemon juiced ⅓ cup high-quality pitted olives

Directions and total time – 1-2 h • COMBINE the paprika, cumin, turmeric, ginger, and cinnamon in a small bowl. Season the chicken thighs generously with salt and pepper on both sides. Rub both sides of each thigh with the spice mixture, using it all. Place in a bowl or plastic bag to marinate for at least 1 hour or up to 3 hours. • ONCE the chicken is done marinating, turn on the Sauté function. Once hot, add the oil. Add 2 of the thighs, skin side down, and cook for about 3 minutes without moving. Remove and repeat with the remaining thighs. Set aside. ● ADD the onion and cook for 2 minutes, scraping the bottom of the pot. Add the garlic and tomato paste and cook, stirring, for 1 more minute. Turn off the Sauté function. Add the broth and scrape any remaining bits off the bottom of the pot. Add the chicken, skin side up, and squeeze them in so that they fit in one layer. Secure the lid. ● COOK at high pressure for 10 minutes and use a natural release. ● REMOVE the chicken and some of the onions. Turn on the Sauté function and simmer the sauce for 10 to 15 minutes, until reduced by more than half and starting to thicken. Turn off the Sauté function. Add the lemon juice, stir, and taste for seasoning. ● TO SERVE, pour the sauce over the chicken and sprinkle the olives on top.

Chicken with Leeks and Mushrooms

Ingredients for 6 servings:

6 chicken breasts boneless and skinless ½ teaspoon Pink Himalayan salt or Celtic Salt ¼ teaspoon pepper 4 tablespoons butter or ghee 3 pounds leeks white and pale green parts only, sliced into circles ½ cup dry white wine or chicken bone broth 1 ¼ pounds cremini mushrooms or button mushrooms, sliced ¼ inch thick 2 tablespoons arrowroot flour ½ cup almond milk plain and unsweetened scallions or fresh parsley to garnish, optional

Directions and total time – 15-30 m • Pat chicken dry and season with salt and pepper. • Set your Instant Pot to the Sauté setting. When hot, heat butter/ghee and brown chicken on both sides. Remove chicken from cooker and transfer to a plate. • Add wine to cooker and deglaze by boiling on sauté setting, stirring and scraping up brown bits, until reduced to about 2 tablespoons, 1 to 2 minutes. • Stir in the wine/broth, leeks and mushrooms. Top the leeks and mushrooms with the chicken breasts and juices from plate. • Using the Manual setting, adjust the Instant Pot to cook on high pressure. Cook for 8 minutes. • When time is up, allow pressure to naturally release for 4 minutes, then release any remaining pressure using the quick release method. • Transfer chicken to a plate. • Stir arrowroot into almond milk and add to Instant Pot returning to sauté setting or on high heat, stirring occasionally, until thickened, about 2 minutes. • Serve chicken on top of leeks and mushrooms.

Zoodle Soup with Chicken

Ingredients for 6 servings:

3 stalks celery diced 2 tbsp pickled jalapeno diced 1 cup bok choy sliced into strips ½ cup fresh spinach 3 Zucchini spiralized 1 tbsp coconut oil ¼ cup button mushrooms diced ¼ medium onion diced 2 cups cooked diced chicken 3 cups chicken broth 1 bay leaf 1 tsp salt ½ tsp garlic powder ⅛ tsp cayenne pepper

Directions and total time – 30-60 m

• Place celery, jalapeno, bok choy, and spinach into medium bowl. Spiralize zucchini; set aside in a separate medium bowl. (The zucchini will not go in the pot during the pressure cooking.) • Press the Sauté button and add the coconut oil to Instant Pot.. Once the oil is hot, add mushrooms and onion. Sauté for 4–6 minutes until onion is translucent and fragrant. Add celery, jalapenos, bok choy, and spinach to Instant Pot. Cook for additional 4 minutes. Press the Cancel button. • Add cooked diced chicken, broth, bay leaf, and seasoning to Instant Pot. Click lid closed. Press the Soup button and set time for 20 minutes. • When timer beeps, allow a 10-minute natural release, and quick-release the remaining pressure. Add spiralized zucchini on Keep Warm mode and cook for additional 10 minutes or until tender. Serve warm.

Chicken Legs with Piquant Mayo Sauce

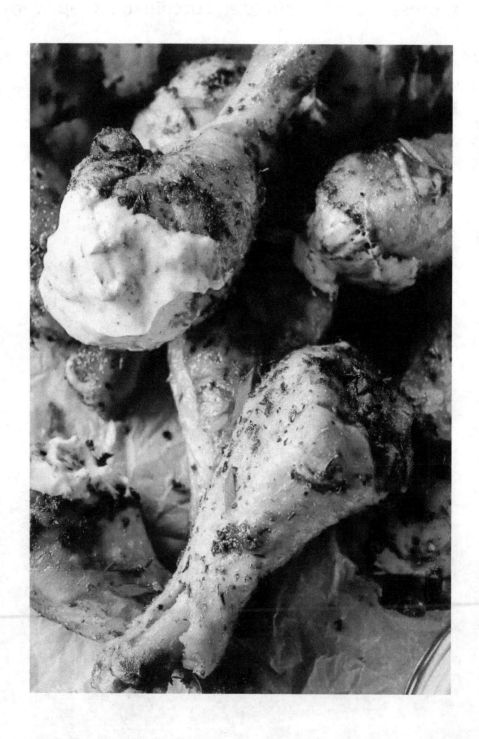

(Ready in about 25 minutes | Servings 4)

Per serving: 484 Calories; 42.6g Fat; 2.4g Carbs; 22.3g Protein; 0.5g Sugars

Ingredients

4 chicken legs, bone-in, skinless 2 garlic cloves, peeled and halved 1/2 teaspoon coarse sea salt 1/4 teaspoon ground black pepper, or more to taste 1/2 teaspoon red pepper flakes, crushed 1 tablespoon olive oil 1/4 cup chicken broth Dipping Sauce: 3/4 cup mayonnaise 2 tablespoons stone ground mustard 1 teaspoon fresh lemon juice 1/2 teaspoon Sriracha Topping: 1/4 cup fresh cilantro, roughly chopped

Directions

Rub the chicken legs with garlic halves; then, season with salt, black pepper, and red pepper flakes. Press the "Sauté" button. Once hot, heat the oil and sauté chicken legs for 4 to 5 minutes, turning once during cooking time. Add a splash of chicken broth to deglaze the bottom of the pan. Secure the lid. Choose "Manual" mode and High pressure; cook for 14 minutes. Once cooking is complete, use a natural pressure release; carefully remove the lid.

Meanwhile, mix all ingredients for the dipping sauce; place in the

refrigerator until ready to serve. Garnish chicken legs with cilantro.

Serve with the piquant mayo sauce on the side. Bon appétit!

Hot Spicy Chicken Soup

(Ready in about 20 minutes | Servings 5)

Per serving: 238 Calories; 17g Fat; 5.4g Carbs; 16.4g Protein; 2.6g Sugars

Ingredients

2 tablespoons grapeseed oil 2 banana shallots, chopped 4 cloves garlic, minced 1 cup Cremini mushrooms, sliced 2 bell peppers, seeded and sliced 1 serrano pepper, seeded and sliced 2 ripe tomatoes, pureed 1 teaspoon porcini powder 2 tablespoons dry white wine Sea salt and ground black pepper, to your liking 1 teaspoon dried basil 1/2 teaspoon dried dill weed 5 cups broth, preferably homemade 4 chicken wings

Directions Press the "Sauté" button and heat the oil. Once hot, sauté the shallots until just tender and aromatic. Add the garlic, mushrooms, and peppers; cook an additional 3 minutes or until softened. Now, stir in tomatoes, porcini powder, white wine, salt, and black pepper. Add the remaining ingredients and stir to combine. Secure the lid. Choose "Manual" mode and High pressure; cook for 18 minutes. Once cooking is complete, use a quick pressure release. Make sure to release any remaining steam and carefully remove the lid. Remove the chicken wings from the Instant Pot. Discard the bones and chop the meat. Add the chicken meat back to the Instant Pot. Ladle into individual bowls and serve warm. Bon appétit!

Chicken Drumsticks in Creamy Butter Sauce

(Ready in about 20 minutes | Servings 6)

Per serving: 351 Calories; 15.7g Fat; 7g Carbs; 43.5g Protein; 3.3g Sugars

Ingredients

2 ripe tomatoes, chopped 1/2 cup roasted vegetable broth, preferably homemade 1 red onion, chopped 1 red bell pepper, seeded and chopped 1 green bell pepper, seeded and chopped 4 cloves garlic 1 teaspoon curry powder 1/2 teaspoon paprika 1/4 teaspoon ground black pepper Sea salt, to taste A pinch of grated nutmeg 1/2 teaspoon ground cumin 2 pounds chicken drumsticks, boneless, skinless 2 tablespoons butter 1/3 cup double cream 1 tablespoon flaxseed meal

Directions

Add tomatoes, vegetable broth, onion, peppers, garlic, curry powder, paprika, black pepper, salt, grated nutmeg, and ground cumin to the bottom of your Instant Pot. Add chicken drumsticks. Secure the lid. Choose "Manual" mode and High pressure; cook for 12 minutes. Once cooking is complete, use a natural pressure release. Allow it to cool completely and reserve the chicken. In a mixing dish, whisk the remaining ingredients and add this mixture to the Instant Pot; press the "Sauté" button and bring it to a boil. Now, add the chicken back to the cooking liquid. Press the "Cancel" button and serve immediately. Bon appétit!

Roasted Turkey Breast Tenderloins

(Ready in about 40 minutes | Servings 6)

Per serving: 255 Calories; 7.1g Fat; 0.7g Carbs; 49.7g Protein; 0g Sugars

Ingredients

6 turkey breast tenderloins 4 cloves garlic, halved 2 tablespoons grapeseed oil 1/2 teaspoon paprika 1/2 teaspoon dried basil 1/2 teaspoon dried oregano 1/2 teaspoon dried marjoram 1 cup water Sea salt, to taste 1/4 teaspoon ground black pepper, or more to taste

Directions

Rub turkey fillets with garlic halves. Now, massage 1 tablespoon of oil into your turkey and season it with paprika, basil, oregano, marjoram, water, salt, and black pepper. Press the "Sauté" button and add another tablespoon of oil. Brown the turkey fillets for 3 to 4 minutes per side. Add the rack to the Instant Pot; lower the turkey onto the rack. Secure the lid. Choose the "Manual" setting and cook for 30 minutes. Once cooking is complete, use a natural pressure release; carefully remove the lid. Serve right away. Bon appétit!

Two-Cheese Chicken Drumsticks

(Ready in about 25 minutes | Servings 5)

Per serving: 409 Calories; 23.8g Fat; 4.8g Carbs; 41.7g Protein; 2.4g Sugars

Ingredients

1 tablespoon olive oil 5 chicken drumsticks 1/2 teaspoon marjoram 1/2 teaspoon thyme 1 teaspoon shallot powder 2 garlic cloves, minced 1/2 cup chicken stock 1/4 cup dry white wine 1/4 cup full-fat milk 6 ounces ricotta cheese 4 ounces cheddar cheese 1/4 teaspoon ground black pepper 1/2 teaspoon cayenne pepper Sea salt, to taste

Directions Press the "Sauté" button and heat the oil. Once hot, brown chicken drumsticks for 3 minutes; turn the chicken over and cook an additional 3 minutes, Now, add marjoram, thyme, shallot powder, garlic, chicken stock, wine, and milk. Secure the lid. Choose the "Manual" setting and cook for 15 minutes. Once cooking is complete, use a natural pressure release; carefully remove the lid. Shred the chicken meat and return to the Instant Pot. Press the "Sauté" button and stir in ricotta cheese, cheddar cheese, black pepper, and cayenne pepper. Cook for a couple of minutes longer or until the cheese melts and everything is heated through. Season with sea salt, taste and adjust the seasonings. Bon appétit!

Greek-Style Chicken Wraps

(Ready in about 20 minutes | Servings 6)

Per serving: 238 Calories; 9.5g Fat; 9.1g Carbs; 29.1g Protein; 6.1g Sugars

Ingredients

1 ½ pounds chicken tenderloin, cut into 1/2-inch pieces Salt and black pepper, to taste 1 teaspoon dried oregano 1/2 teaspoon dried basil 1/2 teaspoon ground cumin 1 cup water 2 ripe tomatoes, pureed 2 garlic cloves, minced 1 tablespoon golden Greek peppers, minced 1 tablespoon freshly squeezed lemon juice 1 large-sized head lettuce 6 ounces Feta cheese, cubed 1 ounce Kalamata olives, pitted and sliced 2 Florina peppers, seeded and chopped

Directions

Add the chicken, salt, black pepper, oregano, basil, cumin, and water to your Instar Pot. Secure the lid. Choose the "Manual" setting and High pressure; cook for 10 minutes. Once cooking is complete, use a natural pressure release; carefully remove the lid. Reserve the chicken. Then, add tomatoes, garlic, and Greek peppers to the Instant Pot. Press the "Sauté" button and cook for 6 minutes at Low pressure. Add the shredded chicken back into the Instant Pot. To serve, divide the chicken mixture among lettuce leaves. Top with Feta cheese, olives, and Florina peppers. Roll up in taco-style, serve and enjoy!

Chicken Fillets with Keto Sauce

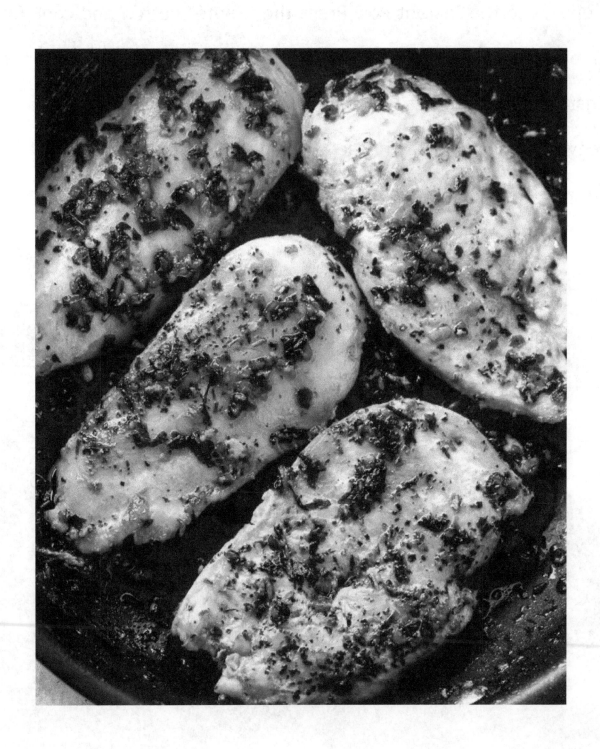

(Ready in about 15 minutes | Servings 4)

Per serving: 314 Calories; 20.3g Fat; 1.7g Carbs; 29.9g Protein; 1.5g Sugars

Ingredients

1 tablespoon peanut oil 1 pound chicken fillets Salt and freshly ground black pepper, to taste 1/2 teaspoon dried basil 1 cup broth, preferably homemade Cheese Sauce: 3 teaspoons butter, at room temperature 1/3 cup double cream 1/3 cup Neufchâtel cheese, at room temperature 1/3 cup Gruyère cheese, preferably freshly grated 3 tablespoons milk 1/2 teaspoon granulated garlic 1 teaspoon shallot powder

Directions

Press the "Sauté" button and add peanut oil. Once hot, sear the chicken fillets for 3 minutes per side. Season the chicken fillets with salt, black pepper, and basil; pour in the broth. Secure the lid. Choose the "Manual" setting and cook for 6 minutes. Once cooking is complete, use a natural pressure release; carefully remove the lid. Clean the Instant Pot and press the "Sauté" button. Now, melt the butter and add double cream, Neufchâtel cheese, Gruyère cheese and milk; add granulated garlic and shallot powder. Cook until everything is heated through. Bon appétit!

Country Chicken Stew

(Ready in about 25 minutes | Servings 6)

Per serving: 453 Calories; 22.6g Fat; 5.9g Carbs; 53.6g Protein; 2.6g Sugars

Ingredients

2 slices bacon 6 chicken legs, skinless and boneless 3 cups water 2 chicken bouillon cubes 1 leek, chopped 1 carrot, trimmed and chopped 4 garlic cloves, minced 1/2 teaspoon dried thyme 1/2 teaspoon dried basil 1 teaspoon Hungarian paprika 1 bay leaf 1 cup double cream 1/2 teaspoon ground black pepper

Directions Press the "Sauté" button to heat up your Instant Pot. Now, cook the bacon, crumbling it with a spatula; cook until the bacon is crisp and reserve. Now, add the chicken legs and cook until browned on all sides. Add the water, bouillon cubes, leeks, carrot, garlic, thyme, basil, paprika, and bay leaf; stir to combine. Secure the lid. Choose the "Poultry" setting and cook for 15 minutes at High pressure. Once cooking is complete, use a natural pressure release; carefully remove the lid. Fold in the cream and allow it to cook in the residual heat, stirring continuously. Ladle into individual bowls, sprinkle each serving with freshly grated black pepper and serve warm. Bon appétit!

Quick and Easy Chicken Carnitas

(Ready in about 20 minutes | Servings 8)

Per serving: 294 Calories; 15.4g Fat; 2.8g Carbs; 35.2g Protein; 1.3g Sugars

Ingredients

3 pounds whole chicken, cut into pieces 3 cloves garlic, pressed 1 guajillo chili, minced 1 tablespoon avocado oil 1/3 cup roasted vegetable broth Sea salt, to taste 1/2 teaspoon ground bay leaf 1/3 teaspoon cayenne pepper 1/2 teaspoon paprika 1/3 teaspoon black pepper 1 cup crème fraiche, to serve 2 heaping tablespoons fresh coriander, chopped

Directions

Place all of the above ingredients, except for crème fraiche and fresh coriander, in the Instant Pot. Secure the lid. Choose the "Poultry" setting and cook for 15 minutes. Once cooking is complete, use a quick pressure release; carefully remove the lid.

Shred the chicken with two forks and discard the bones. Add a dollop of crème fraiche to each serving and garnish with fresh coriander. Enjoy!

Traditional Hungarian Paprikash

(Ready in about 25 minutes | Servings 6

Per serving: 402 Calories; 31.7g Fat; 8.1g Carbs; 21g Protein; 3.4g Sugars

Ingredients

1 tablespoon lard, at room temperature 1 ½ pounds chicken thighs 1/2 cup tomato puree 1 ½ cups water 1 yellow onion, chopped 1 large-sized carrot, sliced 1 celery stalk, diced 2 garlic cloves, minced 2 bell peppers, seeded and chopped 1 Hungarian wax pepper, seeded and minced 1 teaspoon cayenne pepper 1 tablespoon Hungarian paprika 1 teaspoon coarse salt 1/2 teaspoon ground black pepper 1/2 teaspoon poultry seasoning 6 ounces sour cream 1 tablespoon arrowroot powder 1 cup water

Directions

Press the "Sauté" button to heat up the Instant Pot. Now, melt the lard until hot; sear the chicken thighs for 2 to 3 minutes per side. Add the tomato puree, 1 ½ cups of water, onion, carrot, celery, garlic, peppers, and seasonings. Secure the lid. Choose the "Manual" setting and cook for 20 minutes at High pressure. Once cooking is complete, use a quick pressure release; carefully remove the lid. In the meantime, thoroughly combine sour cream, arrowroot powder and 1 cup of water; whisk to combine well. Add the sour cream mixture to the Instant Pot to thicken the cooking liquid. Cook for a couple of minutes on the residual heat. Ladle into individual bowls and serve immediately.

The Best Ever Chicken Goulash

(Ready in about 25 minutes | Servings 6)

Per serving: 353 Calories; 19.5g Fat; 7.5g Carbs; 34.3g Protein; 4.9g Sugars

Ingredients

1 tablespoon olive oil 2 pounds chicken breast halves, boneless and skinless 2 small-sized shallots, chopped 1 teaspoon garlic paste 1 cup milk 2 ripe tomatoes, chopped 1 teaspoon curry powder 1 tablespoon tamari sauce 1 tablespoon balsamic vinegar 2 tablespoons vermouth Sea salt, to taste 1/2 teaspoon cayenne pepper 1/3 teaspoon black pepper 1/2 teaspoon hot paprika 1/2 teaspoon ginger, freshly grated 1 celery stalk with leaves, chopped 1 bell pepper, chopped 1 tablespoon flaxseed meal

Directions Press the "Sauté" button to heat up the Instant Pot. Now, add olive oil. Once hot, sear the chicken breast halves for 3 to 4 minutes per side. Add the shallots, garlic, milk, tomatoes, curry powder, tamari sauce, vinegar, vermouth, salt, cayenne pepper, black pepper, hot paprika, ginger, celery and bell pepper to the Instant Pot; stir to combine well. Secure the lid. Choose the "Meat/Stew" setting and cook for 20 minutes at High pressure. Once cooking is complete, use a quick pressure release; carefully remove the lid. Add flaxseed meal and continue stirring in the residual heat. Ladle into serving bowls and enjoy!

Cheesy Chicken and Mushroom Casserole

(Ready in about 15 minutes | Servings 4)

Per serving: 469 Calories; 32.3g Fat; 8.1g Carbs; 36.3g Protein; 4.2g Sugars

Ingredients

1 tablespoon lard 1 pound chicken breasts, cubed 10 ounces button mushrooms, thinly sliced 2 cloves garlic, smashed 1/2 cup yellow onion, chopped 1/2 teaspoon turmeric powder 1/2 teaspoon shallot powder 1/2 teaspoon dried sage 1/2 teaspoon dried basil Kosher salt, to taste 1/2 teaspoon cayenne pepper 1/3 teaspoon ground black pepper 1 cup chicken broth 1/2 cup double cream 1 cup Colby cheese, shredded

Directions

Press the "Sauté" button to heat up the Instant Pot. Now, melt lard and cook chicken, mushrooms, garlic, and onion; cook until the vegetables are softened. Add turmeric powder, shallot powder, sage, basil, salt, cayenne pepper, black pepper, and broth. Secure the lid. Choose the "Meat/Stew" setting and cook for 6 minutes at High pressure. Once cooking is complete, use a natural pressure release; carefully remove the lid. Now, add double cream and cook in the residual heat until thoroughly heated. Top with cheese and bake in the preheated oven at 390 degrees F until cheese is bubbling. Serve right away.

Chicken Fillets with Sauce

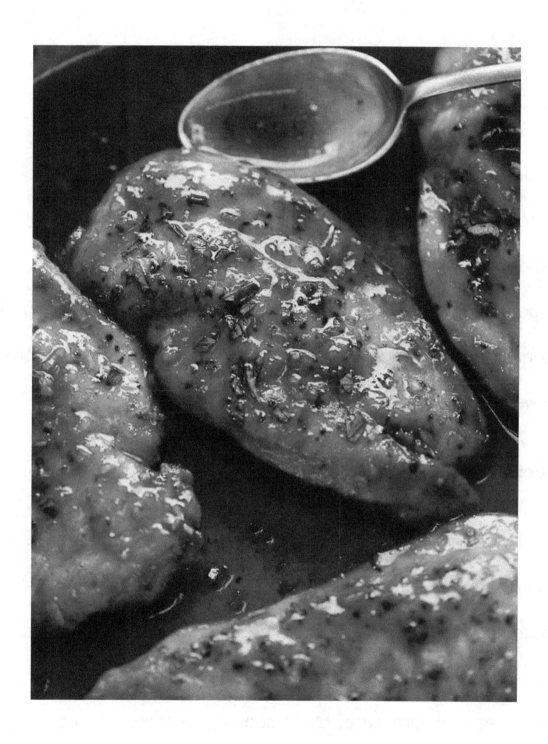

(Ready in about 15 minutes | Servings 8)

Per serving: 109 Calories; 6.5g Fat; 2.3g Carbs; 10g Protein; 0.3g Sugars

Ingredients

1 pound chicken livers 1/2 cup leeks, chopped 2 garlic cloves, crushed 2 tablespoons olive oil 1 tablespoon poultry seasonings 1 teaspoon dried rosemary 1/2 teaspoon dried marjoram 1/4 teaspoon dried dill weed 1/2 teaspoon paprika 1/2 teaspoon red pepper flakes Salt, to taste 1/2 teaspoon ground black pepper 1 cup water 1 tablespoon stone ground mustard

Directions

Press the "Sauté" button to heat up the Instant Pot. Now, heat the oil. Once hot, sauté the chicken livers until no longer pink. Add the remaining ingredients, except for the mustard, to your Instant Pot. Secure the lid. Choose the "Manual" setting and cook for 10 minutes at High pressure. Once cooking is complete, use a quick pressure release; carefully remove the lid. Transfer the cooked

mixture to a food processor; add stone ground mustard. Process

until smooth and uniform. Bon appétit!

Thai Coconut Chicken

(Ready in about 15 minutes | Servings 4

Per serving: 192 Calories; 7.5g Fat; 5.4g Carbs; 25.2g Protein; 2.2g Sugars

Ingredients

1 tablespoon coconut oil 1 pound chicken, cubed 1 shallot, peeled and chopped 2 cloves garlic, minced 1 teaspoon fresh ginger root, julienned 1/3 teaspoon cumin powder 1 teaspoon Thai chili, minced 1 cup vegetable broth, preferably homemade 1 tomato, peeled and chopped 1/3 cup coconut milk, unsweetened 1 teaspoon Thai curry paste 2 tablespoons tamari sauce 1/2 cup sprouts Salt and freshly ground black pepper, to taste

Directions

Press the "Sauté" button to heat up the Instant Pot. Now, heat the coconut oil. Cook the chicken for 2 to 3 minutes, stirring frequently; reserve. Then, in pan drippings, cook the shallot and garlic until softened; add a splash of vegetable broth, if needed. Add ginger, cumin powder and Thai chili and cook until aromatic or 1 minute more. Now, stir in vegetable broth, tomato, coconut milk, Thai curry paste, and tamari sauce. Secure the lid. Choose the "Manual" setting and cook for 10 minutes under High pressure. Once cooking is complete, use a quick pressure release; carefully remove the lid. Afterwards, add sprouts, salt, and black pepper and serve immediately. Bon appétit!

Winter Chicken Salad

(Ready in about 15 minutes + chilling time | Servings 8)

Per serving: 343 Calories; 26.2g Fat; 1.6g Carbs; 24.9g Protein; 0.3g Sugars

Ingredients

2 pounds chicken 1 cup vegetable broth 2 sprigs fresh thyme 1 teaspoon onion powder 1 teaspoon granulated garlic 1/2 teaspoon black pepper, ground 1 bay leaf 1 cup mayonnaise 1 teaspoon Dijon mustard 1 teaspoon fresh lemon juice 2 stalks celery, chopped 2 tablespoons fresh chives, chopped 1/2 teaspoon coarse sea salt

Directions

Place the chicken, broth, thyme, onion powder, garlic, black pepper, and bay leaf in your Instant Pot. Secure the lid. Choose the "Poultry" setting and cook for 12 minutes under High pressure. Once cooking is complete, use a natural pressure release; carefully remove the lid. Remove the chicken from the Instant Pot; allow it to cool slightly. Now, cut the chicken breasts into strips and transfer it to a salad bowl. Add the remaining ingredients and gently stir until everything is well combined. Serve well-chilled and enjoy!

Family Cheese and Chicken Sandwiches

(Ready in about 20 minutes | Servings 4)

Per serving: 500 Calories; 37.4g Fat; 2.2g Carbs; 36.9g Protein; 0.6g Sugars

Ingredients

4 chicken drumsticks, boneless Celery salt, to taste 1/2 teaspoon ground black pepper 1/2 teaspoon cayenne pepper 2 bay leaves 1/3 cup vegetable stock 1 cup water 1/2 cup almond flour 3/4 teaspoon baking powder A pinch of table salt 1/2 teaspoon granulated garlic 2 eggs, whisked 2 tablespoons butter 4 tablespoons mayonnaise 4 teaspoons mustard 4 (1-ounce) slices Cheddar cheese

Directions

Add the chicken drumsticks to the Instant Pot Sprinkle with celery salt, black pepper, and cayenne pepper; add bay leaves, vegetable stock, and water. Now, secure the lid. Choose the "Poultry" setting and cook for 15 minutes under High pressure. Once cooking is complete, use a quick pressure release; carefully remove the lid. Then, mix almond flour with baking powder, table salt, granulated garlic, eggs, and butter in mugs; mix to combine well. Place the mugs in your microwave; microwave for 1 minute 30 seconds on high. Split each roll into halves to make your sandwiches. Assemble your sandwiches with chicken, mayo, mustard and cheese. Serve and enjoy!

Peppery Spicy Ground Chicken

(Ready in about 15 minutes | Servings 6)

Per serving: 231 Calories; 13.6g Fat; 3.1g Carbs; 24.3g Protein; 1.6g Sugars

Ingredients

2 slices bacon, chopped 1 ½ pounds ground chicken 2 garlic cloves, minced 1/2 cup green onions, chopped 1 serrano pepper, chopped 1 red bell pepper, seeded and chopped 1 green bell pepper, seeded and chopped 1 tomato, chopped 1/3 cup chicken broth 1 cup water 1 teaspoon paprika 1/4 teaspoon ground allspice 1 teaspoon onion powder Sea salt and ground black pepper, to taste 2 bay leaves

Directions Press the "Sauté" button to heat up your Instant Pot. Now, cook the bacon until crisp; reserve. Then, brown the ground chicken in bacon grease, crumbling it with a spatula; reserve. Sauté the garlic, green onions, and peppers for 2 to 3 minutes until softened. Stir in the other ingredients. Now, secure the lid. Choose the "Poultry" setting and cook for 5 minutes under High pressure.

Once cooking is complete, use a natural pressure release; carefully

remove the lid. Serve over ketogenic sandwich rolls. Enjoy!

Chicken Legs in Mustard Curry Sauce

(Ready in about 25 minutes | Servings 5)

Per serving: 477 Calories; 26.1g Fat; 4.5g Carbs; 52.8g Protein; 1.4g Sugars

Ingredients

5 chicken legs, boneless, skin-on 2 garlic cloves, halved Sea salt, to taste 1/4 teaspoon black pepper, preferably freshly ground 1/2 teaspoon smoked paprika 2 teaspoons olive oil 1 tablespoon yellow mustard 1 teaspoon curry paste 4 strips pancetta, chopped 1 shallot, peeled and chopped 1 cup roasted vegetable broth, preferably homemade

Directions

Rub the chicken legs with garlic halves; then, season with salt, black pepper, and smoked paprika. Press the "Sauté" button to heat up your Instant Pot. Once hot, heat the oil and sauté chicken legs for 4 to 5 minutes, turning once during cooking. Add a splash of chicken broth to deglaze the bottom of the pan. Spread the legs with mustard and curry paste. Add pancetta, shallot and remaining vegetable broth. Secure the lid. Choose "Manual" mode and High pressure; cook for 14 minutes. Once cooking is complete, use a natural pressure release; carefully remove the lid. Bon appétit!

Budget-Friendly Turkey Salad

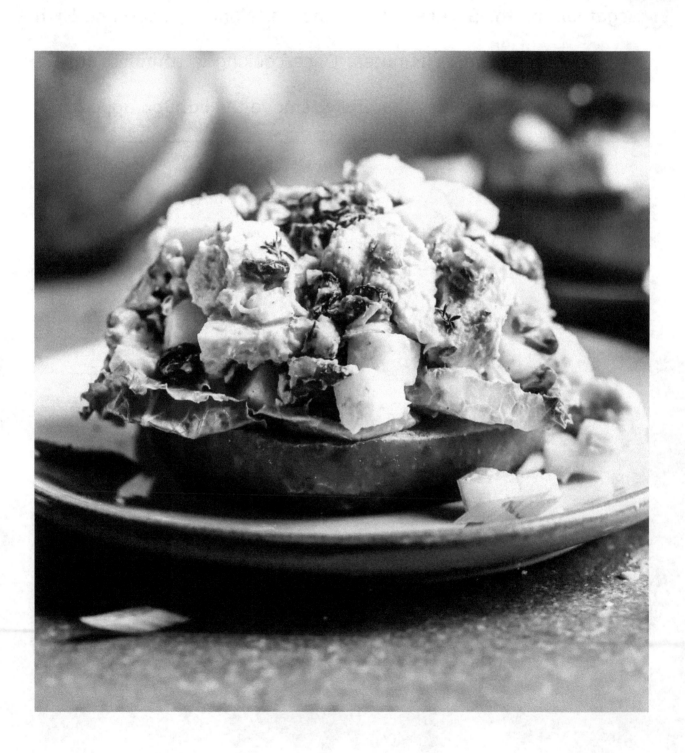

(Ready in about 25 minutes | Servings 6)

Per serving: 321 Calories; 17.2g Fat; 4.4g Carbs; 35g Protein; 1.4g Sugars

Ingredients

2 pounds turkey breast, boneless and skinless 1/2 teaspoon black pepper, preferably freshly ground 1/2 teaspoon red pepper flakes, crushed Seasoned salt, to taste 2 sprigs thyme 1 sprig sage 2 garlic cloves, pressed 1 leek, sliced 1/2 cup mayonnaise 1 ½ tablespoons Dijon mustard 1/2 cup celery, finely diced 1 cucumber, chopped

Directions

Prepare your Instant Pot by adding 1 ½ cups of water and a metal trivet to the bottom of the inner pot. Now, sprinkle turkey breast with black pepper, red pepper, and salt. Lower the seasoned turkey breast onto the trivet. Top with thyme, sage, and garlic. Now, secure the lid. Choose the "Poultry" setting and cook for 20 minutes under High pressure. Once cooking is complete, use a natural pressure release; carefully remove the lid. Allow the turkey to cool completely. Slice the turkey into strips. Add the remaining ingredients and transfer the mixture to a salad bowl. Serve well-chilled. Bon appétit!

Ground Chicken and Zucchini Casserole

(Ready in about 15 minutes | Servings 4)

Per serving: 459 Calories; 32.9g Fat; 6.8g Carbs; 33.8g Protein; 1.8g Sugars

Ingredients

3 teaspoons olive oil 1 pound ground chicken 1/2 cup parmesan cheese, grated 2 tablespoons pork rind crumbs Coarse sea salt and freshly ground black pepper, to taste 2 garlic cloves, minced 1 teaspoon dried basil 1/2 teaspoon dried oregano 1/2 teaspoon dried sage 1/2 pound zucchini, thinly sliced 2 ripe tomatoes, pureed 1/2 cup water 1 teaspoon mustard powder 1 teaspoon minced jalapeño 4 ounces Monterey-Jack cheese, shredded

Directions Press the "Sauté" button to heat up the Instant Pot. Now, heat 1 teaspoon of olive oil until sizzling. Brown ground chicken for 2 minutes, crumbling it with a wide spatula or fork. Now, add parmesan cheese, pork rind crumbs, salt, black pepper, garlic, basil, oregano, and sage. Cook an additional minute and reserve. Wipe down the Instant Pot with a damp cloth; spritz the inner pot with a nonstick cooking spray. Arrange 1/3 of zucchini slices on the bottom. Spread 1/3 of meat mixture over zucchini. Repeat the layering two more times. In a mixing bowl, whisk tomatoes with the remaining 2 teaspoons of olive oil, water, mustard powder, and jalapeno. Pour this tomato sauce over the casserole. Secure the lid. Choose "Manual" mode and High pressure; cook for 10 minutes. Once cooking is complete, use a quick pressure release; carefully remove the lid. Then, top the casserole with shredded cheese; allow it to melt on the residual heat. Bon appétit

---

Saucy Chicken Drumettes with Squashsta

(Ready in about 55 minutes | Servings 8)

Per serving: 224 Calories; 9.4g Fat; 7g Carbs; 26.4g Protein; 1.1g Sugars

Ingredients

2 tablespoons grapeseed oil 8 chicken drumettes 2 cloves garlic, minced Sea salt and ground black pepper, to taste 2 ripe tomatoes, pureed 2 tablespoons capers, rinsed and drained 1 cup broth, preferably homemade 1 tablespoon flaxseed meal 1 (3-pound) spaghetti squash, halved 1 tablespoon olive oil Coarse sea salt, to taste

Directions

Press the "Sauté" button to heat up the Instant Pot. Heat the grapeseed oil. Brown the chicken drumettes for 2 to 3 minutes per side. Add the garlic, salt, black pepper, tomatoes, capers, and broth. Secure the lid. Choose "Manual" mode and High pressure;

cook for 10 minutes. Once cooking is complete, use a natural pressure release; carefully remove the lid. Reserve the chicken drumettes. Press the "Sauté" button again and add the flaxseed meal to the Instant Pot. Thicken the tomato sauce for a couple of minutes or until your desired thickness is achieved. Preheat your oven to 380 degrees F. Place squash halves, cut-side down on a lightly greased baking pan. Drizzle olive oil over them and sprinkle with sea salt. Roast for 40 minutes. Afterwards, scrape the flesh to create "spaghetti". Serve with warm chicken drumettes and tomato sauce. Enjoy!

Two-Cheese Turkey Bake

(Ready in about 30 minutes | Servings 8)

Per serving: 472 Calories; 33g Fat; 3.2g Carbs; 38.9g Protein; 0.7g Sugars

Ingredients

2 pounds turkey breasts 2 garlic cloves, halved Sea salt and ground black pepper, to taste 1 teaspoon paprika 1 tablespoon butter 10 slices Colby cheese, shredded 2/3 cup mayonnaise 1/3 cup sour cream 1 cup Romano cheese, preferably freshly grated

Directions

Rub the turkey breast with garlic halves; now, sprinkle with salt, black pepper, and paprika. Press the "Sauté" button to heat up the Instant Pot. Melt the butter and sear the turkey breast for 2 to 3 minutes per side. In a mixing bowl, combine shredded Colby cheese, mayonnaise, sour cream, 1/2 cup of grated Romano. Spread this mixture over turkey breast; top with the remaining

Romano cheese. Secure the lid. Choose "Manual" mode and High pressure; cook for 20 minutes. Once cooking is complete, use a quick pressure release; carefully remove the lid. Bon appétit!

Easy One-Pot Mexican Chili

(Ready in about 35 minutes | Servings 6)

Per serving: 391 Calories; 27g Fat; 8.1g Carbs; 28.4g Protein; 4.9g Sugars

Ingredients

1 tablespoon olive oil 1 pound turkey, ground 1/2 pound pork, ground 1 onion, finely chopped 2 garlic cloves, minced 2 ripe tomatoes, pureed 1 Mexican chili pepper, minced 1/2 teaspoon ground cumin 1 teaspoon red pepper flakes Salt and ground black pepper, to taste 1 cup chicken stock 1 ½ cups Mexican cheese blend

Directions

Press the "Sauté" button to heat up the Instant Pot. Heat the olive oil and brown the turkey and pork until no longer pink or about 3 minutes. Add the remaining ingredients, except for Mexican cheese blend, to your Instant Pot. Secure the lid. Choose "Poultry" mode and High pressure; cook for 15 minutes. Once cooking is complete, use a natural pressure release; carefully remove the lid. Ladle into soup bowls; top each bowl with Mexican cheese blend and serve hot.

Turkey Breasts with Homemade Pesto

(Ready in about 25 minutes | Servings 6)

Per serving: 391 Calories; 26.3g Fat; 1.8g Carbs; 34.9g Protein; 0.4g Sugars

Ingredients

2 pounds turkey breast Sea salt and ground black pepper, to taste 1 teaspoon paprika 1 tablespoon olive oil 1 cup water Pesto Sauce: 2 tablespoons pine nuts, toasted 1/2 cup fresh basil leaves 1/3 cup Parmesan cheese, grated 1/3 cup olive oil 1 garlic clove, halved Salt and ground black pepper, to taste

Directions

Season turkey breast with salt, black pepper, and paprika. Press the "Sauté" button to heat up the Instant Pot. Heat 1 tablespoon of olive oil and sear the turkey breast for 2 to 3 minutes per side. Pour in the water and secure the lid. Choose "Poultry" mode and High pressure; cook for 20 minutes. Once cooking is complete, use a quick pressure release; carefully remove the lid. To make the pesto sauce, add the pine nuts and fresh basil leaves to your food processor. Add the remaining ingredients and process until everything is well incorporated. Serve the prepared turkey breast with pesto sauce. Bon appétit!

Holiday Chicken Wrapped in Prosciutto

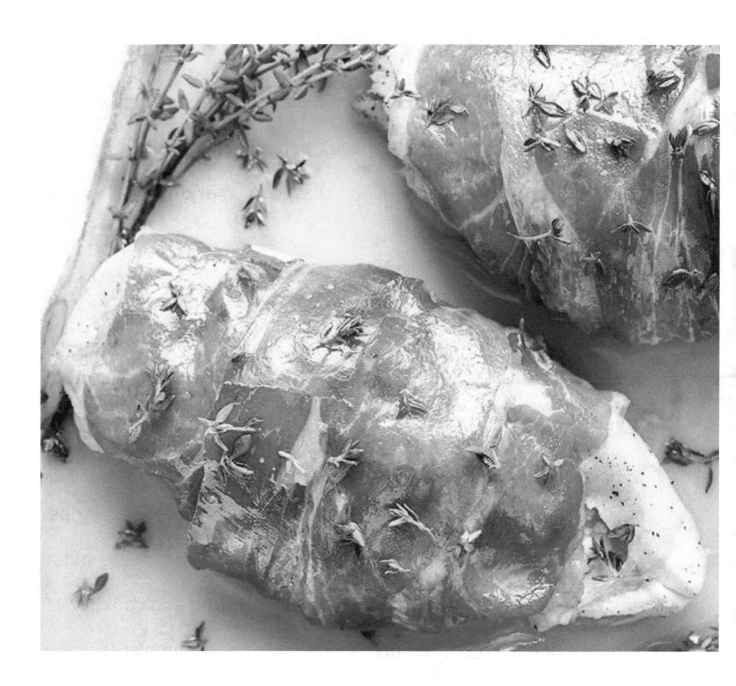

(Ready in about 20 minutes | Servings 5)

Per serving: 548 Calories; 28.4g Fat; 1.1g Carbs; 68.3g Protein; 0g Sugars

Ingredients

5 chicken breast halves, butterflied 2 garlic cloves, halved Sea salt, to taste 1/4 teaspoon ground black pepper, or more to taste 1/2 teaspoon red pepper flakes 1 teaspoon marjoram 10 strips prosciutto

Directions

Prepare the Instant Pot by adding 1 ½ cups of water and metal trivet to the bottom. Rub chicken breast halves with garlic. Then, season the chicken with salt, black pepper, red pepper, and marjoram. Then, wrap each chicken breast into 2 prosciutto strips; secure with toothpicks. Arrange wrapped chicken on the metal trivet. Secure the lid. Choose the "Poultry" setting and cook for 15 minutes under High pressure. Once cooking is complete, use a natural pressure release; carefully remove the lid. Bon appétit!

Moroccan Chicken Wraps

Ingredients for 6 servings:

1 cup roasted red peppers drained 1 tsp ground coriander 1 tsp ground cumin 1 tsp garlic powder ½ tsp ground chipotle pepper ½ tsp caraway seeds ½ cup Water 1 lb boneless skinless chicken thighs trimmed of fat ¼ tsp salt ¾ cup plain 2% Greek yogurt ½ cup chopped fresh mint ⅓ cup finely chopped red onion 6 light flour tortillas heated in a skillet until slightly charred 1 lemon cut into 6 wedges

Directions and total time – 30-60 m

• Combine the peppers, coriander, cumin, garlic powder, chipotle, caraway, and water in a blender. Secure the lid and purée until smooth. • Place the chicken thighs in the Instant Pot. Top with the puréed pepper mixture. Seal the lid, close the valve, and set the Manual/Pressure Cook button to 10 minutes. • Use a natural pressure release for 10 minutes, followed by a quick pressure release. When the valve drops, carefully remove the lid. Remove the chicken with a slotted spoon and place on a cutting board. Let the chicken stand for 5 minutes before shredding. • Press the Cancel button and set to Sauté. Then press the Adjust button to "More" or "High." Bring to a boil and boil for 5 minutes to thicken slightly. Stir the chicken and salt into the sauce. • In a medium bowl, combine the yogurt, mint, and onion. Spoon the yogurt mixture evenly over each tortilla, squeeze the lemon wedges over each serving, and top with equal amounts of the chicken mixture. Fold the edges of the tortillas over or serve open face with a knife and fork, if desired.

Conclusion

Thank you for making it throughout, it would certainly be nice to have feedback of your sensations regarding these quick dishes to remain in shape without having to give up the satisfaction of eating your favored meals.

Keep in mind that this diet does not just aim at slendering however also at physical health, look for the best way to trigger your metabolic rate, and keep in mind that this diet plan routine is a genuine anti-aging routine, the recipes in this book will allow you to have fun as well as drop weight at the same time and this will certainly permit you to slim down in a calm and loosened up means without needing to reduce yourself to a circumstance of anxiety and also frustration.

Enjoy as well as appreciate your diet regimen.

CPSIA information can be obtained
at www.ICGtesting.com
Printed in the USA
BVHW060159250621
610373BV00007B/1712